Herbal Remedies for 20 Common Ailments

TABLEOF CONTENTS

- Resources for Further Learning and Exploration

CHAPTER 1

HEADACHES AND MIGRAINES

1.1 Peppermint, Lavender, and Feverfew: Nature's Headache Relievers

Peppermint (Mentha piperita):

Properties: Peppermint contains menthol, which is known for its soothing and muscle relaxant properties. It can help alleviate tension headaches and improve blood circulation.

Preparation:

1. Boil a cup of water.

2. Place 1-2 teaspoons of dried peppermint leaves (or 1 peppermint tea bag) in a cup.

3. Pour the boiling water over the peppermint.

4. Cover the cup and let it steep for about 10 minutes.

5. Strain the tea, and sip it slowly.
Note:You can also inhale the steam from your cup while sipping the tea for added relief.

Lavender (Lavandulaangustifolia):

Properties: Lavender has calming and anti-inflammatory properties. It's particularly useful for tension headaches caused by stress and anxiety.

<u>Preparation</u>:

1. Boil a cup of water.

2. Place 1-2 teaspoons of dried lavender flowers (or 1 lavender tea bag) in a cup.

3. Pour the boiling water over the lavender.

4. Cover the cup and steep for about 5-7 minutes.

5. Strain the teaand enjoy.

Feverfew (Tanacetum parthenium):

<u>Properties</u>: Feverfew helps reduce the frequency and intensity of migraines by inhibiting blood vessel consriction and inflammation.

<u>Preparation</u>:

<u>Note</u>: Consult a healthcare professional for theappropriate dosageand preparation method for feverfew. It's often taken as a daily supplement or used in tincture form.

1.2 Herbal Teas and Compresses for Soothing Head Pain

Peppermint Tea:

<u>Preparation</u>:

1. Boil a cup of water.

2. Place 1-2 teaspoons of dried peppermint leaves (or 1 peppermint tea bag) in a cup.

3. Pour the boiling water over the peppermint.

4. Cover the cup and let it steep for about 10 minutes.

5. Strain the tea, and sip it slowly.

Lavender Compress:

<u>Preparation</u>:

1. Boil a cup of water.

2. Place 1-2 teaspoons of dried lavender flowers (or 1 lavender tea bag) in a cup.

3. Pour the boiling water over the lavender.

4. Cover the cup and steep for about 5-7 minutes.

5. Strain the tea, then soak a clean cloth or towel in it.

6. Wring out theexcess liquid and apply the warm, damp cloth to your forehead for soothing relief.

Feverfew Tincture:

<u>Preparation:</u>

<u>Note</u>: Consult a healthcare professional or herbalist for guidanceon using feverfew tincture. They can recommend theappropriate dosageand usage instructions.

CHAPTER 2

INSOMNIA AND SLEEP DISORDERS

2.1 Chamomile, Valerian, and Passionflower: Herbal Sleep Aids

Chamomile (Matricaria chamomilla):

Properties: Chamomile has mild sedative properties and is known for its ability to promote relaxation and improve sleep quality.

Preparation:

1. Boil a cup of water.

2. Place 1-2 teaspoons of dried chamomile flowers (or 1 chamomile tea bag) in a cup.

3. Pour the boiling water over the chamomile.

4. Cover the cup and steep for about 5-7 minutes.

5. Strain the tea, and enjoy it before bedtime.

Valerian (Valerianaofficinalis):

Properties: Valerian is a potent sedativeand muscle relaxant. It can help you fall asleep faster and improve theoverall quality of your sleep.

Preparation:

1. Valerian is available in various forms, including capsules, tablets, and tinctures.

2. Follow the recommended dosage instructions on the product packaging. It's typically taken 30 minutes to 1 hour before bedtime.

Passionflower (Passiflora incarnata):

<u>Properties</u>: Passionflower has calming and anxiety-reducing effects, making it helpful for those whoexperience sleep disturbances due to stress.

<u>Preparation:</u>

1. Boil a cup of water.

2. Place 1-2 teaspoons of dried passionflower leaves and flowers (or 1 passionflower tea bag) in a cup.

3. Pour the boiling water over the passionflower.

4. Cover the cup and steep for about 10 minutes.

5. Strain the tea, and sip it about an hour before bedtime.

2.2 Creating a Relaxing Bedtime Routine with Herbs

Herbal Sleep Tea:

<u>Preparation:</u>

1. Combineequal parts of dried chamomile, valerian, and passionflower.

2. Boil a cup of water.

3. Place 1-2 teaspoons of the herbal blend in a cup.

4. Pour the boiling water over the herbs.

5. Cover the cup and steep for about 10 minutes.

6. Strain the teaand enjoy it as part of your calming bedtime routine.

Aromatherapy with Lavender:

<u>Preparation:</u>

1. Usea diffuser to disperse lavender essential oil into your bedroom.

2. Alternatively, dilute lavender essential oil with a carrier oil (e.g., coconut oil) and use it for a soothing massage before sleep. Apply a small amount to your temples, wrists, and the soles of your feet.

Valerian Capsules:

<u>Preparation:</u>

1. Purchase valerian capsules from a reputable source.

2. Follow the recommended dosage instructions on the product packaging. Take them 30 minutes to 1 hour before bedtime.

Make sure toconsulta healthcare professional or herbalist for personalized advice, especially if you have underlying health conditions or are taking medications.

CHAPTER 3

STRESS AND ANXIETY

3.1 Lemon Balm, Ashwagandha, and Holy Basil: Herbs for Relaxation

Lemon Balm (Melissaofficinalis):

Properties: Lemon balm is a calming herb that can reduce stress and anxiety, promote relaxation, and improve mood.

Preparation:

1. Boil a cup of water.

2. Place 1-2 teaspoons of dried lemon balm leaves (or 1 lemon balm tea bag) in a cup.

3. Pour the boiling water over the lemon balm.

4. Cover the cup and steep for about 10 minutes.

5. Strain the teaand sip it throughout the day.

Ashwagandha (Withania somnifera):

Properties: Ashwagandha is an adaptogenic herb that helps the body adapt to stress and restore balance.

Preparation:

1. Ashwagandha is commonly available in powder or capsule form.

2. Follow the recommended dosage instructions on the product packaging. It's typically taken onceor twicea day with meals.

Holy Basil (Ocimum sanctum):

<u>Properties</u>: Holy basil, also known as tulsi, has adaptogenic and anxiolytic properties, helping to reduce stress and anxiety.

<u>Preparation</u>:

1. Boil a cup of water.

2. Place 1-2 teaspoons of dried holy basil leaves (or 1 holy basil tea bag) in a cup.

3. Pour the boiling water over the holy basil.

4. Cover the cup and steep for about 5-7 minutes.

5. Strain the teaand enjoy it multiple times a day.

3.2 Herbal Tinctures and Aromatherapy for Anxiety Relief

Lemon Balm Tincture:

<u>Preparation</u>:

1. Purchasea lemon balm tincture from a reputable source.

2. Follow the recommended dosage instructions on the product packaging. Usually, it's taken in drop form diluted in water or juice.

Aromatherapy with Lavender:

<u>Preparation</u>:

1. Usea diffuser to disperse lavender essential oil into your surroundings.

2. Alternatively, you can dilute lavender essential oil with a carrier oil and use it for a calming massage. Apply it to your pulse points or takea relaxing bath with a few drops added to the water.

CHAPTER 4

DIGESTIVE UPSET

4.1 Ginger, Peppermint, and Fennel: Herbal Allies for the Stomach

Ginger (Zingiber officinale):

Properties: Ginger is well-known for its anti-nauseaand digestive properties. It helps alleviate indigestion and soothean upset stomach.

Preparation:

1. Peel and slice fresh ginger (about a 1-inch piece).

2. Boil a cup of water and add the ginger slices.

3. Simmer for 5-10 minutes.

4. Strain the ginger teaand sip it slowly.

Peppermint (Mentha piperita):

Properties: Peppermint is a natural digestiveaid, known for relieving gas, bloating, and indigestion.

Preparation:

1. Boil a cup of water.

2. Place 1-2 teaspoons of dried peppermint leaves (or 1 peppermint tea bag) in a cup.

3. Pour the boiling water over the peppermint.

4. Cover the cup and steep for about 10 minutes.

5. Strain the teaand enjoy it after meals.

Fennel (Foeniculum vulgare):

Properties: Fennel is excellent for relieving digestive discomfort, including gas and bloating.

Preparation:

1. Boil a cup of water.

2. Crush 1-2 teaspoons of fennel seeds using a mortar and pestle.

3. Place the crushed seeds in a cup and pour the boiling water over them.

4. Cover the cup and steep for about 10 minutes.

5. Strain the teaand sip it slowly.

4.2 Herbal Bitters and Digestive Tonics for Improved Digestion

Herbal Bitters:

Preparation:

1. You can purchase herbal bitters from a storeor make your own using a combination of bitter herbs such as dandelion root, gentian, and burdock.

2. Follow the recommended dosage instructions on the product packaging or the recipe provided.

CHAPTER 5

COMMON COLDS AND FLU

5.1 Echinacea, Elderberry, and Garlic: Boosting Immunity Naturally

Echinacea (Echinacea purpurea):

Properties: Echinacea is an immune-boosting herb that can help prevent and reduce the severity of colds and flu.

Preparation:

1. Echinacea is available in various forms, including capsules, tinctures, and teas.

2. Follow the recommended dosage instructions on the product packaging. Start taking it at the first sign of illness.

Elderberry (Sambucus nigra):

Properties:Elderberry is rich in antioxidants and can help reduce the duration and severity of cold and flu symptoms.

Preparation:

1. Elderberry syrup or elderberry extract is readily available in stores. Follow the recommended dosage instructions on the product packaging.

Garlic (Allium sativum):

<u>Properties:</u> Garlic has natural antiviral and antibacterial properties, making it an excellent addition to your diet during cold and flu season.

<u>Preparation:</u>

1. Incorporate fresh garlic into your meals regularly.

2. Consider taking garlic supplements following the recommended dosage instructions on the product packaging.

5.2 Herbal Soups and Infusions for Cold and Flu Relief

Herbal Chicken Soup:

<u>Preparation:</u>

1. Preparea chicken soup with added immune-boosting herbs such as echinacea, thyme, and garlic.

2. Simmer the soup for an extended period toextract the herbs' medicinal properties.

3. Consume the soup regularly toalleviate cold and flu symptoms.

Thymeand Honey Infusion:

<u>Preparation:</u>

1. Boil a cup of water.

2. Place 1-2 teaspoons of dried thyme leaves (or 1 thyme tea bag) in a cup.

3. Pour the boiling water over the thyme.

4. Cover the cup and steep for about 5-7 minutes.

5. Strain the tea, add a spoonful of honey, and drink it while warm. Thymeand honey help soothea sore throat and cough.

CHAPTER 6

SORE THROAT

6.1 Marshmallow Root, Sage, and Slippery Elm: Soothing Soreness

Marshmallow Root (Althaeaofficinalis)

<u>Properties:</u> Marshmallow root contains mucilage that coats the throat and provides soothing relief from soreness.

<u>Preparation:</u>

1. Boil a cup of water.

2. Place 1-2 teaspoons of dried marshmallow root (or 1 marshmallow root tea bag) in a cup

CHAPTER 7

ALLERGIES

7.1 Nettle, Butterbur, and Quercetin: Natural Antihistamines

Nettle (Urtica dioica):

Properties: Nettle is a natural antihistamineand anti-inflammatory herb, which can alleviateallergy symptoms like sneezing and itching.

Preparation:

1. Boil a cup of water.

2. Place 1-2 teaspoons of dried nettle leaves (or 1 nettle tea bag) in a cup.

3. Pour the boiling water over the nettle.

4. Cover the cup and steep for about 5-7 minutes.

5. Strain the teaand drink it throughout the day.

Butterbur (Petasites hybridus)

Properties: Butterbur has antihistamineand anti-inflammatory properties, making it effective in reducing allergy symptoms.

Preparation:

1. Butterbur is commonly available in capsuleor tablet form.

2. Follow the recommended dosage instructions on the product packaging.

Quercetin:

Properties: Quercetin is a natural flavonoid found in foods likeonions and apples. It acts as a natural antihistamineand anti-inflammatory.

Preparation:

1. Quercetin supplements areavailable in stores. Follow the recommended dosage instructions on the product packaging.

7.2 Herbal Steam Inhalations and Allergy Teas

Herbal Steam Inhalation:

Preparation:

1. Boil a pot of water.

2. Add a handful of dried nettle leaves or chamomile flowers.

3. Place your faceover the pot (not too close toavoid burns) and inhale the steam deeply.

4. You can alsoadd a drop of eucalyptus or peppermint essential oil toenhance the inhalation.

Allergy Tea Blend:

Preparation:

1. Combineequal parts of dried nettle, chamomile, and elderflower.

2. Boil a cup of water.

3. Place 1-2 teaspoons of the herbal blend in a cup.

4. Pour the boiling water over the herbs.

5. Cover the cup and steep for about 10 minutes.

6. Strain the teaand sip it several times a day during allergy season.

CHAPTER 8

ARTHRITIS AND JOINT PAIN

8.1 Turmeric, Boswellia, and Willow Bark: Anti-Inflammatory Herbs

Turmeric (Curcuma longa)

Properties: Turmeric contains curcumin, a potent anti-inflammatory compound that can help reduce joint pain and inflammation.

Preparation:

1. Createa turmeric paste by mixing turmeric powder with a small amount of water.

2. Apply the paste to theaffected joints and let it sit for 15-20 minutes before rinsing.

Boswellia (Boswellia serrata):

Properties: Boswellia is a natural anti-inflammatory that can help relieve joint pain and improve mobility.

Preparation:

1. Boswellia is often available in capsuleor tablet form.

2. Follow the recommended dosage instructions on the product packaging.

Willow Bark (Salix spp.):

Properties: Willow bark contains salicin, a natural pain reliever and anti-inflammatory compound, similar toaspirin.

Preparation:

1. Boil a cup of water.

2. Place 1-2 teaspoons of dried willow bark (or 1 willow bark tea bag) in a cup.

3. Pour the boiling water over the willow bark.

4. Cover the cup and steep for about 10 minutes.

5. Strain the teaand drink it for pain relief.

8.2 Topical Herbal Balms and Joint Massage Techniques

Herbal Balm for Joint Pain:

Preparation:

1. Combine melted coconut oil with a few drops of essential oils like lavender or eucalyptus.

2. Add a teaspoon of powdered turmeric and mix well.

3. Allow the mixture to solidify at room temperature.

4. Apply the balm to theaffected joints and gently massage.

Joint Massage Techniques:

<u>Preparation</u>:

1. Perform gentle joint massage using warm coconut oil infused with a few drops of essential oils like ginger or frankincense.

2. Use circular motions and light pressure to soothe theaffected joints.

CHAPTER 9

HIGH BLOOD PRESSURE

9.1 Hawthorn, Garlic, and Olive Leaf: Herbs for Heart Health

Hawthorn (Crataegus spp.):

Properties: Hawthorn is a cardiac tonic that can help improve heart function and lower blood pressure.

Preparation:

1. Boil a cup of water.

2. Place 1-2 teaspoons of dried hawthorn berries (or 1 hawthorn tea bag) in a cup.

3. Pour the boiling water over the hawthorn.

4. Cover the cup and steep for about 10 minutes.

5. Strain the teaand drink it daily.

Garlic (Allium sativum):

Properties: Garlic has natural blood pressure-lowering properties and can improveoverall heart health.

Preparation:

1. Incorporate fresh garlic into your meals regularly.

2. Consider taking garlic supplements following the recommended dosage instructions on the product packaging.

Olive Leaf (Oleaeuropaea):

Properties:Olive leaf extract has cardiovascular benefits and can help lower blood pressure.

Preparation:

1. Olive leaf extract is commonly available in liquid or capsule form.

2. Follow the recommended dosage instructions on the product packaging.

9.2 Herbal Recipes and Lifestyle Tips for Hypertension

Hawthorn Berry Smoothie:

Preparation:

1. Blend a handful of fresh or frozen berries with a banana, yogurt, and a teaspoon of dried hawthorn berries.

2. Enjoy this heart-healthy smoothie regularly.

Garlic-Roasted Vegetables:

Preparation:

1. Toss mixed vegetables in oliveoil and minced garlic.

2. Roast until tender and season with herbs like rosemary and thyme for added flavor.

<u>Lifestyle Tips:</u>

1. Adopt a low-sodium diet rich in whole grains, fruits, and vegetables.

2. Engage in regular exercise, such as brisk walking or swimming.

3. Practice stress-reduction techniques like yogaor meditation.

CHAPTER 10

DIABETES MANAGEMENT

10.1 Cinnamon, Fenugreek, and Gymnema: Herbs for Blood Sugar Control

Cinnamon (Cinnamomum verum)

Properties: Cinnamon can help improve insulin sensitivity and regulate blood sugar levels.

Preparation:

1. Add a pinch of cinnamon to your morning coffee, tea, or oatmeal.

2. Consider cinnamon supplements following the recommended dosage instructions on the product packaging.

Fenugreek (Trigonella foenum-graecum):

Properties:Fenugreek seeds contain soluble fiber and compounds that can help lower blood sugar levels.

Preparation:

1. Soak fenugreek seeds overnight and consume them in the morning.

2. Fenugreek supplements arealsoavailable. Follow the recommended dosage instructions on the product packaging.

Gymnema (Gymnema sylvestre):

<u>Properties:</u> Gymnema can reduce sugar cravings and improve blood sugar control.

<u>Preparation:</u>

1. Gymnema supplements areavailable in various forms. Follow the recommended dosage instructions on the product packaging.

10.2 Incorporating Herbs into Diabetic-Friendly Meals

Cinnamon-Spiced Sweet Potatoes:

<u>Preparation:</u>

1. Roast sweet potato chunks with a sprinkleof cinnamon for a delicious and blood sugar-friendly side dish.

Fenugreek Salad:

<u>Preparation:</u>

1. Sprinkle fenugreek seeds on top of salads for added flavor and blood sugar benefits.

Lifestyle Tips:

1. Monitor blood sugar levels regularly.

2. Maintain a balanced diet with a focus on low-glycemic foods.

3. Engage in regular physical activity to help control blood sugar.

Note: Consulta healthcare professional before making significant dietary or supplement changes, especially if readers have underlying health conditions or are taking medications.

CHAPTER 11

SKIN CONDITIONS (ACNE, ECZEMA, PSORIASIS)

11.1 Calendula, Tea Tree, and Aloe Vera: Skin-Soothing Herbs

Calendula (Calendulaofficinalis):

Properties: Calendula has anti-inflammatory and antimicrobial properties, making it effective for soothing skin irritations and promoting healing.

Preparation:

1. Infused CalendulaOil:

   - Place dried calendula flowers in a clean glass jar.

   - Cover the flowers with a carrier oil likeoliveoil or coconut oil.

   - Seal the jar and place it in a sunny spot for 2-4 weeks, shaking it daily.

   - Strain theoil, and it's ready for use.

2. Apply the infused oil topically toaffected areas or add a few drops to your bathwater.

Tea Tree (Melaleucaalternifolia):

Properties: Tea treeoil is well-known for its antimicrobial and anti-inflammatory properties, making it effectiveagainst acneand fungal skin conditions.

<u>Preparation</u>:

1. Diluted Tea TreeOil:

- Mix a few drops of tea treeessential oil with a carrier oil (e.g., jojobaor sweet almond oil).

- Apply the diluted mixture toaffected areas using a cotton ball or swab.

- Avoid using undiluted tea treeoil on the skin as it can be too strong.

AloeVera (Aloe barbadensis miller):

<u>Properties</u>:Aloe vera is known for its soothing and healing properties, making it ideal for relieving burns, eczema, and dry skin.

<u>Preparation</u>:

1. Fresh Aloe Vera Gel:

- Cut a maturealoe vera leaf and extract the gel.

- Apply the gel directly to theaffected area.

2. Commercial Aloe Vera Products:

- Purchasealoe vera gel or cream from a reputable source.

- Apply the product to theaffected skin as directed on the packaging.

It is important to do patch testing beforeapplying any new herbal remedy toa larger areaof the skin and it is recommended to seek advice from a dermatologist for severeor chronic skin conditions.

CHAPTER 12

RESPIRATORY HEALTH

12.1 Thyme, Eucalyptus, and Mullein: Respiratory Relief Herbs

Thyme (Thymus vulgaris):

Properties: Thyme is rich in thymol, an antimicrobial compound that helps relieve respiratory congestion and soothe coughs.

Preparation:

1. Boil a cup of water.

2. Place 1-2 teaspoons of dried thyme leaves (or 1 thyme tea bag) in a cup.

3. Pour the boiling water over the thyme.

4. Cover the cup and steep for about 10 minutes.

5. Strain the tea, add honey for taste, and sip it toease congestion.

Eucalyptus (Eucalyptus globulus)

Properties:Eucalyptus essential oil is a potent decongestant and expectorant, helping to clear airways.

Preparation:

1. Add a few drops of eucalyptus essential oil toa bowl of hot water.

2. Inhale the steam by covering your head with a towel and leaning over the bowl.

Mullein (Verbascum thapsus):

<u>Properties:</u> Mullein helps soothe irritation in the respiratory tract and reduce coughing.

<u>Preparation:</u>

1. Boil a cup of water.

2. Place 1-2 teaspoons of dried mullein leaves (or 1 mullein tea bag) in a cup.

3. Pour the boiling water over the mullein.

4. Cover the cup and steep for about 10 minutes.

5. Strain the teaand drink it toease coughs and congestion.

12.2 Herbal Steam Inhalations and Chest Rubs for Respiratory Support

Herbal Steam Inhalation:

<u>Preparation:</u>

1. Boil a pot of water.

2. Add a handful of dried thyme leaves or eucalyptus leaves.

3. Place your faceover the pot (not too close toavoid burns) and inhale the steam deeply to relieve congestion.

Chest Rub with Eucalyptus:

<u>Preparation:</u>

1. Mix a few drops of eucalyptus essential oil with a carrier oil (e.g., coconut oil).

2. Gently rub the mixtureon your chest and throat before bed to promoteeasy breathing.

CHAPTER 13

DIGESTIVE HEALTH

13.1 Dandelion, Ginger, and Peppermint: Digestive Helpers

Dandelion (Taraxacum officinale):

<u>Properties</u>: Dandelion stimulates digestion, improves appetite, and supports liver health.

<u>Preparation</u>:

1. Boil a cup of water.

2. Place 1-2 teaspoons of dried dandelion root (or 1 dandelion tea bag) in a cup.

3. Pour the boiling water over the dandelion.

4. Cover the cup and steep for about 10 minutes.

5. Strain the teaand drink it before meals toaid digestion.

Ginger (Zingiber officinale):

<u>Properties</u>: Ginger promotes digestion and alleviates nauseaand indigestion.

<u>Preparation</u>:

1. Peel and slice fresh ginger (about a 1-inch piece).

2. Boil a cup of water and add the ginger slices.

3. Simmer for 5-10 minutes.

4. Strain the ginger teaand sip it slowly after meals.

Peppermint (Mentha piperita):

Properties: Peppermint is a natural digestiveaid, known for relieving gas, bloating, and indigestion.

Preparation:

1. Boil a cup of water.

2. Place 1-2 teaspoons of dried peppermint leaves (or 1 peppermint tea bag) in a cup.

3. Pour the boiling water over the peppermint.

4. Cover the cup and steep for about 10 minutes.

5. Strain the teaand enjoy it after meals.

13.2 Herbal Bitters and Digestive Tonics for Better Digestion

Herbal Bitters:

Preparation:

1. You can purchase herbal bitters from a storeor make your own using a combination of bitter herbs such as dandelion root, gentian, and burdock.

2. Follow the recommended dosage instructions on the product packaging or the recipe provided.

CHAPTER 14

SLEEP DISORDERS

14.1 Valerian, Lavender, and Chamomile: Herbal Sleep Aids

Valerian (Valerianaofficinalis):

Properties: Valerian is a potent sedative that can help with insomniaand anxiety-related sleep issues.

Preparation:

1. Valerian is often available in capsuleor tablet form.

2. Follow the recommended dosage instructions on the product packaging.

Lavender (Lavandulaangustifolia):

Properties: Lavender has calming and anti-inflammatory properties, making it ideal for promoting sleep.

Preparation:

1. Boil a cup of water.

2. Place 1-2 teaspoons of dried lavender flowers (or 1 lavender tea bag) in a cup.

3. Pour the boiling water over the lavender.

4. Cover the cup and steep for about 5-7 minutes.

5. Strain the teaand enjoy it before bedtime.

Chamomile (Matricaria chamomilla):

<u>Properties</u>: Chamomile is a gentle sedativeand relaxant, making it ideal for promoting sleep.

<u>Preparation</u>:

1. Boil a cup of water.

2. Place 1-2 teaspoons of dried chamomile flowers (or 1 chamomile tea bag) in a cup.

3. Pour the boiling water over the chamomile.

4. Cover the cup and steep for about 5-7 minutes.

5. Strain the teaand enjoy it before bedtime.

14.2 Creating a Relaxing Bedtime Routine with Herbs

Herbal Sleep Tea:

<u>Preparation</u>:

1. Combineequal parts of dried valerian, lavender, and chamomile.

2. Boil a cup of water.

3. Place 1-2 teaspoons of the herbal blend in a cup.

4. Pour the boiling water over the herbs.

5. Cover the cup and steep for about 10 minutes.

6. Strain the teaand enjoy it as part of your calming bedtime routine.

Aromatherapy with Lavender:

<u>Preparation</u>:

1. Usea diffuser to disperse lavender essential oil into your bedroom.

2. Alternatively, dilute lavender essential oil with a carrier oil (e.g., coconut oil) and use it for a relaxing massage before sleep. Apply a small amount to your temples, wrists, and the soles of your feet.

CHAPTER 15

ANXIETY AND STRESS RELIEF

15.1 Lemon Balm, Ashwagandha, and Passionflower: Nature's Stress Relievers

Lemon Balm (Melissaofficinalis):

<u>Properties:</u> Lemon balm is a calming herb that can reduce stress and anxiety, promote relaxation, and improve mood.

<u>Preparation:</u>

1. Boil a cup of water.

2. Place 1-2 teaspoons of dried lemon balm leaves (or 1 lemon balm tea bag) in a cup.

3. Pour the boiling water over the lemon balm.

4. Cover the cup and steep for about 10 minutes.

5. Strain the teaand sip it throughout the day.

Ashwagandha (Withania somnifera):

<u>Properties:</u>Ashwagandha is an adaptogenic herb that helps the body adapt to stress and restore balance.

<u>Preparation:</u>

1. Ashwagandha is commonly available in powder or capsule form.

2. Follow the recommended dosage instructions on the product packaging. It's typically taken onceor twicea day with meals.

Passionflower (Passiflora incarnata)

Properties: Passionflower is a natural sedativeand anxiolytic herb that can help reduceanxiety and induce calmness.

Preparation:

1. Boil a cup of water.

2. Place 1-2 teaspoons of dried passionflower leaves and stems (or 1 passionflower tea bag) in a cup.

3. Pour the boiling water over the passionflower.

4. Cover the cup and steep for about 10 minutes.

5. Strain the teaand enjoy it when feeling anxious or stressed.

15.2 Herbal Tinctures and Aromatherapy for Anxiety Relief

Lemon Balm Tincture:

Preparation:

1. Purchasea lemon balm tincture from a reputable source.

2. Follow the recommended dosage instructions on the product packaging. Usually, it's taken in drop form diluted in water or juice.

Ashwagandha Tincture:

<u>Preparation:</u>

1. Purchasean ashwagandha tincture from a reputable source.

2. Follow the recommended dosage instructions on the product packaging.

Aromatherapy with Lavender:

<u>Preparation:</u>

1. Usea diffuser to disperse lavender essential oil into your surroundings.

2. Alternatively, you can dilute lavender essential oil with a carrier oil (e.g., coconut oil) and use it for a calming massage. Apply it to your pulse points or takea relaxing bath with a few drops added to the water.

Consulta healthcare professional, especially if you have severeanxiety or stress-related issues, as these herbs may interact with certain medications or medical conditions.

CHAPTER 16

IMMUNE SUPPORT

16.1 Echinacea, Elderberry, and Astragalus: Immune-Boosting Herbs

Echinacea (Echinacea purpurea):

Properties:Echinacea is an immune-boosting herb that can help prevent and reduce the severity of colds and flu.

Preparation:

1. Echinacea is available in various forms, including capsules, tinctures, and teas.

2. Follow the recommended dosage instructions on the product packaging. Start taking it at the first sign of illness.

Elderberry (Sambucus nigra):

Properties:Elderberry is rich in antioxidants and can help reduce the duration and severity of cold and flu symptoms.

Preparation:

1. Elderberry syrup or elderberry extract is readily available in stores. Follow the recommended dosage instructions on the product packaging.

Astragalus (Astragalus membranaceus):

Properties:Astragalus is an adaptogenic herb that supports immune health and helps the body resist infections.

Preparation:

1. Boil a cup of water.

2. Place 1-2 teaspoons of dried astragalus root (or 1 astragalus tea bag) in a cup.

3. Pour the boiling water over theastragalus.

4. Cover the cup and steep for about 10 minutes.

5. Strain the teaand drink it regularly to boost immunity.

16.2 Herbal Soups and Immune Tonic Recipes

Immune-Boosting Soup:

Preparation:

1. Preparea vegetable soup with added immune-boosting herbs such as echinacea, thyme, and garlic.

2. Simmer the soup for an extended period toextract the herbs' medicinal properties.

3. Consume the soup regularly during cold and flu season.

Elderberry Immune Tonic:

<u>Preparation:</u>

1. Combineelderberry syrup with a few drops of echinacea tincture.

2. Take this immune-boosting tonic daily to support your body's defenses.

CHAPTER 17

HEADACHES AND MIGRAINES

17.1 Feverfew, Peppermint, and Lavender: Herbal Allies for Headache Relief

Feverfew (Tanacetum parthenium):

Properties: Feverfew is known for its ability to reduce the frequency and severity of migraines.

Preparation:

1. Chew on fresh feverfew leaves daily.

2. You can also take feverfew supplements following the recommended dosage instructions on the product packaging.

Peppermint (Mentha piperita):

Properties: Peppermint has a calming effect on headaches and can alleviate tension and migraine-related symptoms.

Preparation:

1. Boil a cup of water.

2. Place 1-2 teaspoons of dried peppermint leaves (or 1 peppermint tea bag) in a cup.

3. Pour the boiling water over the peppermint.

4. Cover the cup and steep for about 10 minutes.

5. Strain the teaand sip it to relieve headaches.

Lavender (Lavandulaangustifolia):

Properties: Lavender is known for its soothing and calming properties, which can help alleviate headache pain.

Preparation:

1. Boil a cup of water.

2. Place 1-2 teaspoons of dried lavender flowers (or 1 lavender tea bag) in a cup.

3. Pour the boiling water over the lavender.

4. Cover the cup and steep for about 5-7 minutes.

5. Strain the teaand sip it toease headache discomfort.

17.2 Herbal Compresses and Aromatherapy for Headache Relief

Peppermint Compress:

Preparation:

1. Brew a strong cup of peppermint tea.

2. Soak a clean cloth in the warm tea.

3. Place the damp cloth on your forehead and relax for 15-20 minutes.

Aromatherapy with Lavender:

<u>Preparation</u>:

1. Usea diffuser to disperse lavender essential oil into your surroundings.

2. Alternatively, dilute lavender essential oil with a carrier oil (e.g., jojobaor almond oil) and massage it into your temples and neck toease headache tension.

CHAPTER 18

WOMEN'S HEALTH (MENSTRUAL CRAMPS AND MENOPAUSE)

18.1 Chaste Tree Berry, Black Cohosh, and Ginger: Women's Health Allies

Chaste Tree Berry (Vitex agnus-castus):

Properties: Chaste tree berry is used to relieve symptoms of PMS and regulate the menstrual cycle.

Preparation:

1. Chaste tree berry is available in capsuleor tincture form.

2. Follow the recommended dosage instructions on the product packaging.

Black Cohosh (Actaea racemosa):

Properties: Black cohosh is known for its ability toalleviate menopausal symptoms such as hot flashes and mood swings.

Preparation:

1. Black cohosh is available in capsules or tinctures.

2. Follow the recommended dosage instructions on the product packaging.

Ginger (Zingiber officinale):

Properties: Ginger can help reduce menstrual cramps and alleviate nauseaassociated with PMS.

Preparation:

1. Peel and slice fresh ginger (about a 1-inch piece).

2. Boil a cup of water and add the ginger slices.

3. Simmer for 5-10 minutes.

4. Strain the ginger teaand sip it toease menstrual discomfort.

18.2 Herbal Teas and Lifestyle Tips for Women's Health

Chaste Tree Berry Tea:

Preparation:

1. Boil a cup of water.

2. Place 1-2 teaspoons of dried chaste tree berries (or 1 chaste tree berry tea bag) in a cup.

3. Pour the boiling water over the chaste tree berries.

4. Cover the cup and steep for about 10 minutes.

5. Strain the teaand drink it daily to support menstrual regularity.

Lifestyle Tips:

1. Maintain a healthy diet rich in fruits, vegetables, and whole grains.

2. Engage in regular physical activity to manage PMS and menopausal symptoms.

3. Consider stress reduction techniques like yogaor meditation to support overall well-being.

CHAPTER 19

SKIN HEALTH (ACNE, ECZEMA, PSORIASIS)

19.1 Calendula, Tea Tree, and Aloe Vera: Skin-Soothing Herbs

Calendula (Calendulaofficinalis):

<u>Properties</u>: Calendula has anti-inflammatory and antimicrobial properties, making it effective for soothing skin irritations and promoting healing.

<u>Preparation</u>:

1. Infused CalendulaOil:

   - Place dried calendula flowers in a clean glass jar.

   - Cover the flowers with a carrier oil likeoliveoil or coconut oil.

   - Seal the jar and place it in a sunny spot for 2-4 weeks, shaking it daily.

   - Strain theoil, and it's ready for use.

2. Apply the infused oil topically toaffected areas or add a few drops to your bathwater.

Tea Tree (Melaleucaalternifolia):

<u>Properties</u>: Tea treeoil is a potent decongestant and expectorant, helping to clear airways.

<u>Preparation</u>:

1. Add a few drops of tea treeessential oil toa bowl of hot water.

2. Inhale the steam by covering your head with a towel and leaning over the bowl.

AloeVera (Aloe barbadensis miller):

Properties:Aloe vera is known for its soothing and healing properties, making it ideal for relieving burns, eczema, and dry skin.

Preparation:

1. Fresh Aloe Vera Gel:

   - Cut a maturealoe vera leaf and extract the gel.

   - Apply the gel directly to theaffected area.

2. Commercial Aloe Vera Products:

   - Purchasealoe vera gel or cream from a reputable source.

   - Apply the product to theaffected skin as directed on the packaging.

It is important to consulta healthcare professional before making significant dietary or supplement changes, especially if you have underlying health conditions or are taking medications.

CHAPTER 20

STRESS AND ANXIETY RELIEF

20.1 Lemon Balm, Ashwagandha, and Chamomile: Natural Stress Busters

Lemon Balm (Melissaofficinalis):

Properties: Lemon balm is a calming herb that can reduce stress and anxiety, promote relaxation, and improve mood.

Preparation:

1. Boil a cup of water.

2. Place 1-2 teaspoons of dried lemon balm leaves (or 1 lemon balm tea bag) in a cup.

3. Pour the boiling water over the lemon balm.

4. Cover the cup and steep for about 10 minutes.

5. Strain the teaand sip it throughout the day.

Ashwagandha (Withania somnifera):

Properties:Ashwagandha is an adaptogenic herb that helps the body adapt to stress and restore balance.

Preparation:

1. Ashwagandha is commonly available in powder or capsule form.

2. Follow the recommended dosage instructions on the product packaging. It's typically taken onceor twicea day with meals.

Chamomile (Matricaria chamomilla):

<u>Properties</u>: Chamomile is a gentle sedativeand relaxant, making it ideal for reducing stress and anxiety.

<u>Preparation</u>:

1. Boil a cup of water.

2. Place 1-2 teaspoons of dried chamomile flowers (or 1 chamomile tea bag) in a cup.

3. Pour the boiling water over the chamomile.

4. Cover the cup and steep for about 5-7 minutes.

5. Strain the teaand enjoy it when feeling anxious or stressed.

20.2 Herbal Tinctures and Aromatherapy for Stress Relief

Lemon Balm Tincture:

<u>Preparation:</u>

1. Purchasea lemon balm tincture from a reputable source.

2. Follow the recommended dosage instructions on the product packaging. Usually, it's taken in drop form diluted in water or juice.

Ashwagandha Tincture:

<u>Preparation:</u>

1. Purchasean ashwagandha tincture from a reputable source.

2. Follow the recommended dosage instructions on the product packaging.

Aromatherapy with Chamomile:

<u>Preparation:</u>

1. Usea diffuser to disperse chamomileessential oil into your surroundings.

2. Alternatively, dilute chamomileessential oil with a carrier oil (e.g., coconut oil) and use it for a relaxing massageor add a few drops to your bath for stress relief.

CONCLUSION

Herbal remedies offer a natural and time-tested approach to improving your health and well-being. Throughout this e-book, we'veexplored a wide rangeof herbs and their applications for common ailments. Hereare some key takeaways:

1. *Consult a Professional*: Before incorporating any new herbal remedy into your routine, itsessential to consult with a healthcare professional, especially if you have underlying health conditions or are taking medications.

2. *Quality Matters*: Choose high-quality herbs and herbal products from reputable sources toensureeffectiveness and safety.

3. *Start Slowly:*When using herbal supplements, start with lower doses and gradually increase them as needed while monitoring for any adverse reactions.

4. *Consistency is Key*: Many herbal remedies work best with consistent useover time. Incorporate them into your daily routine for optimal benefits.

5. *Holistic Approach*: Herbal remedies are most effective when combined with a healthy lifestyle, including a balanced diet, regular exercise, and stress management techniques.

6. *Listen to Your Body*: Pay attention to how your body responds to herbal remedies. Adjust your approach if needed and be patient with the healing process.

Remember that herbs are not a replacement for medical treatment when necessary. They can complement conventional medicineand help maintain overall health.

By exploring and embracing the world of herbal remedies, you can take chargeof your health and well-being in a natural and empowering way.